FROM MANAGING TO CONQUERING ILEOSTOMY

Expert Guide To Understanding the Causes, Recognizing Symptoms, Prevention and Embracing Effective Treatments for a Vibrant and Healthy Life

DR. DASHIELL DANIEL

CHAPTER ONE   18

CHAPTER TWO   23

CHAPTER THREE   30

CHAPTER FOUR   34

Disclaimer

This book, is intended to provide information and guidance on the subject matter and is not a substitute for professional medical advice, diagnosis, or treatment.

The author does not own or endorse any such entities mentioned in the book. Any resemblance to actual persons, living or dead, or actual events is purely coincidental.

Readers are encouraged to consult with qualified healthcare professionals for medical advice, diagnosis, and treatment tailored to their specific circumstances.

The author and the publisher disclaim any liability for any loss or risk, personal or otherwise, arising directly or indirectly from the use of the information presented in this book.

By reading this book, the reader acknowledges and agrees to the terms of this disclaimer.

"Ileostomy: Navigating Life's New Path" is a priceless tool for people dealing with the significant life adjustments brought about by ileostomy surgery. Carefully crafted by combining medical knowledge with human understanding, this all-encompassing manual explores the core concepts of ileostomy and offers a road map for people to adjust, overcome obstacles, and enjoy happy, fulfilling lives after surgery.

The preface extends a hearty welcome to readers, expressing gratitude for their participation and outlining the goals of the book. The credentials of the author serve as further evidence of the reliability of the information provided, guaranteeing that readers are well-informed and guided by an informed source. The main body of the book delves into the fundamentals of ileostomy, explaining its definition, types, and the medical justification for the procedure. Surgical procedures are deconstructed, providing readers with a more profound comprehension of the interventions that transform their lives.

Chapter 2 thoughtfully addresses the emotional and psychological aspects of adjusting to change, recognizing the significant impact on people's lives. Coping mechanisms, lifestyle modifications, and the importance of support networks are examined, offering a comprehensive approach to recovery. Chapter 3 dives into the day-to-day necessities with necessary supplies and equipment, providing guidance on selecting the appropriate appliances and guaranteeing appropriate upkeep and care.

"Daily Management Techniques" (Chapter 4) provides readers with a comprehensive guide to managing their daily routines by covering essential topics such as stoma care, dietary considerations, and hygiene practices. Chapter 5 addresses challenges, such as managing odor and dealing with leakage and skin irritation, enabling readers to confront these issues with confidence.

Chapter 6 promotes physical activity and exercise, highlighting customized routines and the role of sports and recreational activities in maintaining a healthy lifestyle.

Chapter 7 delves into the social aspects of living with an ileostomy, covering communication, intimacy, and dispelling stigma and misconceptions. Chapter 8 offers practical advice for work and career planning, highlighting workplace accommodations and the careful balancing act between health and career goals.

In Chapter 9, the book adopts a forward-looking perspective, examining future innovations and research in ostomy care. This section informs readers about the changing landscape of ileostomy care, covering topics such as patient advocacy and technological advancements.

The book's final chapter, "Inspiring Success Stories," puts the human element front and center, with profiles and first-hand accounts of ileostomy champions who overcame obstacles to provide hope to those starting their own journeys.

With its blend of clinical expertise, useful advice, and inspirational narratives, "Ileostomy: Navigating Life's New Path" is more than just a book—it's a lifeline for people navigating the challenges of life after ileostomy. It fosters resilience and gives people the confidence and optimism to embrace their new paths.

Overview

As we set out on this journey to conquer ileostomy, we must first extend a warm welcome to those who are looking for help and direction in overcoming the obstacles presented by this surgical intervention. This exploration dives into the nuances of living with an ileostomy, providing support, guidance, and helpful advice for people adjusting to this life-altering change.

The author acknowledges the importance of this journey and, with this comprehensive guide, hopes to serve as a useful tool for patients as well as healthcare professionals who care for people with ileostomies.

Knowledge About Ileostomy

Understanding the ileostomy surgical procedure is essential to overcoming it. An ileostomy is when the last segment of the small intestine, the ileum, is diverted to an opening made on the abdomen called a stoma. This rerouting of the digestive tract requires the use of an external pouching system to collect waste, which changes the excretory process. Understanding the anatomy and physiology of this procedure is essential for people to understand the functional changes and successfully adjust to the new reality imposed by an ileostomy.

Getting Used To Physical Shifts

Managing the physical changes resulting from an ileostomy is a crucial part of the process of overcoming this procedure. Patients will need to adjust to their new abdominal appearance as well as the practical aspects of managing the stoma and pouching system.

This section covers topics like stoma care, hygiene, and the selection of appropriate ostomy products. It also provides helpful advice and techniques for preserving skin health around the stoma, selecting suitable pouching systems, and resolving common problems. These will enable individuals to face the physical adjustments with confidence and competence.

Psychosocial Repercussions

It is impossible to overstate the psychosocial effects of having an ileostomy because people struggle with a wide range of emotions, from acceptance and resilience to anxiety and grief. In order to achieve overall well-being, it is imperative to comprehend and address the psychological aspects of having an ileostomy. This section will discuss the emotional journey and provide guidance on coping mechanisms, support systems, and mental health strategies.

It will also address the impact of body image and self-esteem and offer guidance on fostering a positive self-perception and cultivating resilience in the face of the psychosocial challenges associated with ileostomy.

Nutritional Aspects

Overcoming ileostomy requires a sophisticated grasp of dietary factors in order to maximize health and wellness. The surgically created new anatomy impacts the digestive system and nutritional absorption, requiring dietary adjustments.

This section explains the dietary adjustments necessary in order to control output consistency, avoid dehydration, and minimize potential complications. Useful advice on meal planning, hydration, and navigating food choices enables people to make decisions that support their nutritional needs and improve their quality of life in general.

Exercise And Physical Activity

Remaining active and healthy is essential to overcoming ileostomy and enhancing overall health. This section discusses the adjustments and modifications needed to exercise and engage in physical activity with an ileostomy.

From selecting suitable exercises to addressing issues like stoma protection and preventing hernias during physical exertion, this section offers a thorough guide to integrating fitness into the lives of people with ileostomies. By busting myths and providing useful guidance, it hopes to boost self-assurance and promote the many advantages of continuing to be active after ileostomy.

Handling Closeness And Bonds In Partnerships

The effect of ileostomy on intimacy and relationships is a sensitive and frequently disregarded aspect of life after surgery.

This section discusses the emotional and physical aspects of intimacy, providing advice on self-esteem, communication, and adjusting to changes in sexual function. It also looks at ways to encourage open communication with partners, bust myths, and maintain healthy relationships after ileostomy. By recognizing and addressing these intimate aspects, people can deal with the complexities of relationships in a more resilient and understanding way.

Collaboration in Healthcare and Support from Professionals

Together, the patient and a multidisciplinary healthcare team must work together to conquer ileostomy. This section highlights the value of professional support, including the roles of dietitians, ostomy nurses, mental health specialists, and surgeons in providing holistic care. It also discusses the significance of regular follow-up appointments, ongoing education, and monitoring for potential complications to provide patients with the knowledge and tools they need to succeed over the long term. Working together with healthcare professionals is essential to conquering ileostomy because it guarantees a thorough and customized approach to treatment.

overcoming an ileostomy is a complex process that involves physical, psychological, and practical aspects. Through comprehension of the surgical process, adjustment to physical changes, psychosocial support, dietary management, physical activity integration, intimacy and relationship management, and working in conjunction with healthcare providers, people can empower themselves to lead happy, healthy lives after an ileostomy. This extensive manual is an invaluable tool for anyone starting this process because it provides encouragement, understanding, and useful guidance to help them overcome obstacles and seize chances for development and resiliency.

CHAPTER ONE
FUNDAMENTALS OF ILEOSTOMIA

A surgical procedure called an ileostomy entails making an opening in the abdomen called a stoma that connects to the small intestine. Ileostomies are commonly performed when the flow of digestive waste needs to be diverted away from the colon and rectum. Ileostomies are often indicated in cases where the lower digestive tract is compromised or diseased, necessitating the bypass of certain sections of the bowel.

The main goal of an ileostomy is to enable the direct passage of bodily waste—specifically, gas and stool—through the stoma and into an external collection pouch. This surgical intervention has a significant impact on the individual's digestive process, and patients and healthcare providers must have a thorough understanding of its implications.

Ileostomy Definition And Types

Ileostomies can be categorized into various types based on their specific anatomical locations and surgical techniques. The most common types are end ileostomy, loop ileostomy, and continent ileostomy. An end ileostomy is a surgical procedure in which the end of the small intestine is brought through the abdominal wall to form a stoma, whereas a loop ileostomy is a surgical procedure in which a loop of the small intestine is created through the abdominal wall, forming two openings—one for stool and one for mucus. Continent ileostomies, on the other hand, use a surgically constructed pouch within the body to collect waste, which must be periodically emptied by the patient. Each type of ileostomy has unique considerations, benefits, and challenges, depending on the underlying medical condition and the specific goals of the surgical procedure.

Ileostomy For Medical Reasons

Ileostomies are performed for a variety of medical reasons, most frequently in response to conditions that impact the health or functionality of the lower digestive system. Inflammatory bowel diseases (IBD), which include Crohn's disease and ulcerative colitis, are common indications for ileostomies. These conditions involve chronic inflammation of the gastrointestinal tract and result in symptoms like severe abdominal pain, diarrhea, and complications like strictures or fistulas. In some cases, colorectal cancer may require the removal of portions of the colon or rectum, making an ileostomy an essential part of the treatment regimen. Other medical reasons for ileostomies include trauma or injuries to the bowel, congenital abnormalities, or refractory infections.

Surgical Techniques

The creation of an ileostomy begins with the identification of the appropriate anatomical site for the stoma on the abdominal wall. This decision is influenced by factors such as the patient's anatomy, lifestyle considerations, and the underlying medical condition. The surgical team must make sure that the stoma placement allows for optimal pouching, minimizing the risk of complications like leakage or irritation. After the stoma is established, the surgeon either creates a temporary diversion (in the case of loop ileostomy) or disconnects the colon and rectum entirely.

The closure of the ileum to of

Patients undergoing ileostomy care require ongoing postoperative care. Healthcare providers educate patients on stoma care, including cleaning techniques, applying appliances correctly, and keeping an eye out for any signs of infection or irritation. Dietary adjustments may be required to account for the changes in digestive function, and patients typically go through an adjustment period to get used to the physical and psychological aspects of living with an ileostomy. Long-term follow-up is critical to address any complications that may arise, such as stoma prolapse, retraction, or herniation. Patients with conditions like IBD or colorectal cancer also require regular surveillance because ongoing monitoring helps detect any recurrence or progression of the underlying disease.

the ideas related to ileostomy cover a wide range of topics, from the basic knowledge of the procedure and its varieties to the medical justifications for its use and the complexities of the surgical procedures that are involved. A thorough understanding of these ideas is essential for medical professionals who provide care for patients who have ileostomies, as well as for patients who are navigating the psychological and physical difficulties that come with this surgical intervention. With continued education, support, and advancements in surgical techniques, the management of ileostomies will continue to develop, enhancing the general health and quality of life for those who have this life-changing procedure.

CHAPTER TWO
CHANGE-ADVANTING

The process of adjusting to the major lifestyle changes brought about by an ileostomy is complex and calls for perseverance, determination, and optimism. Patients who have ileostomy surgery notice a significant change in their daily routines, physical capacities, and self-perception.

This adjustment affects many areas of life, such as personal hygiene, nutrition, and social interactions. In the area of personal hygiene, patients must learn and master the skills related to managing an ostomy pouch, making sure that it is applied correctly and changing it on a regular basis to avoid complications. Additionally, adjusting to dietary changes is vital because some foods may affect the function of the ileostomy and require cautious and thoughtful nutrition.

In addition to the physical changes, adjusting to an ileostomy has a significant psychological impact. Managing the changed perception of one's body, possible feelings of shame, and navigating how society views ostomy patients can be difficult. In order to effectively address these emotional aspects, individuals must receive counseling or psychotherapy. Support groups and peer networks are also essential for facilitating adaptation as they provide a forum for people to share experiences, trade coping mechanisms, and create a sense of community. Healthcare professionals, such as nurses and psychologists, also play a vital role in this adaptation process by offering information, direction, and emotional support.

Handling The Emotional Effect

The psychological effects of having an ileostomy are a significant factor that require careful thought and focused interventions. Patients may experience a variety of emotions, such as anxiety, depression, and a sense of loss. The change in body image and the worry about possible stigmatization can lead to a lower quality of life. Coping mechanisms include a mix of psychological support, education, and building resilience. Mental health providers are essential in assisting individuals in navigating these emotional challenges by offering a secure environment in which to express feelings and anxieties.

In addition, it is critical to incorporate psychosocial support into the healthcare framework. Patients can connect with other individuals going through similar experiences through support groups designed specifically for ileostomy patients, which promotes a feeling of community and mutual understanding. Patients can also be empowered to deal with emotional challenges head-on by receiving education about the surgical procedure, possible complications, and the overall impact on daily life. Finally, patients can benefit from an environment where concerns can be promptly addressed by healthcare providers, which promotes emotional well-being. Managing the emotional impact of ileostomy patients ultimately calls for a comprehensive strategy that takes into account both the psychological state of the individual and their social support networks.

Modifications To Lifestyle

The lifestyle changes that come with having an ileostomy surgery are significant and affect many aspects of a person's day-to-day life. Patients have to adjust to these changes, which range from activity limitations to dietary changes, in order to maximize their overall quality of life. Dietary changes are especially important in order to avoid complications like blockages or irritation around the stoma. People who have an ileostomy frequently have to be more careful about what they eat, with an emphasis on eating a balanced diet that reduces the risk of dehydration and electrolyte imbalances.

In addition to dietary considerations, people need to modify their wardrobe choices to cover up the ostomy pouch. This may entail trying on various outfits, learning where to put the pouch optimally, and making sure that ostomy accessories are secure and comfortable. People also need to stay hydrated because ileostomy can result in increased fluid loss. As such, people should be cautious about how much fluid they drink, especially in circumstances where dehydration could be a concern.

To protect the stoma and avoid potential injuries, lifestyle modifications are required when it comes to physical activity. While regular exercise is recommended, extreme abdominal strain or impact should be avoided. Physiotherapists and other healthcare professionals are essential in helping patients with appropriate exercise recommendations and ensuring a gradual return to physical activity.

Resources And Support Systems

Creating strong support networks and getting access to pertinent resources are essential steps on the path to conquering ileostomy. Patients going through this life-changing experience gain a great deal from having a support system consisting of medical professionals, friends, family, and other ostomates. Medical professionals are the main source of knowledge, direction, and medical expertise, providing constant monitoring and assistance during the adaptation process. Follow-up appointments allow medical professionals to address any new issues that may arise, evaluate the patient's progress, and make any required modifications to the treatment plan.

Family and friends are an important source of the emotional and practical support that people with an ileostomy need. Their comprehension, support, and participation in the process of adaptation enhance the patient's overall quality of life. Online and offline educational resources are a great source of information about living with an ileostomy; they cover topics like pouch care, dietary guidelines, and emotional well-being. Additionally, ostomy support groups and organizations give people a place to connect, exchange stories, and gain insightful knowledge from others who have successfully navigated similar obstacles.

When it comes to employment and social integration, it is crucial to have access to resources that encourage inclusivity and awareness. People who have an ileostomy could benefit from accommodations at work, and campaigns to dispel myths and lessen stigma can create a more accepting community. To sum up, creating a strong support system and making use of the resources that are available are crucial steps toward enabling people to overcome the obstacles that come with having an ileostomy and lead happy, fulfilling lives.

CHAPTER THREE
ESSENTIAL SUPPLIES AND EQUIPMENT

Gaining control over ileostomy necessitates a thorough comprehension of the necessary supplies and equipment that are integral to the day-to-day management of this condition. Among the basic supplies is the ostomy pouch, which gathers waste and comes in different styles, such as one-piece or two-piece systems. Moreover, skin barriers or wafers form a seal around the stoma, shielding the skin from irritation brought on by digestive enzymes. Odor-control products, adhesive removers, and wipes are essential for preserving hygiene and avoiding skin problems. Lastly, accessories like belts and covers improve the comfort and discreteness of the ostomy pouch, fostering a sense of normalcy in the lives of those who have ileostomy. Knowledge of these supplies and equipment is essential for conquering ileostomy.

Overview Of Products For Ostomies

A thorough understanding of ostomy products is essential for anyone dealing with the challenges of having an ileostomy. These products range widely and are made to help people live a comfortable and functional life after surgery. In addition to pouching systems, barriers, and adhesives, ostomy products also include colostomy irrigation systems, specialized ostomy belts for added security, and deodorizing products to address odor concerns. More recent innovations include ostomy products that are equipped with cutting-edge technologies, like sensors that can monitor pouch capacity. With this knowledge, people are better able to make decisions based on their unique needs and preferences, which ultimately improves their quality of life after ileostomy surgery.

Selecting Appropriate Appliances

Choosing the appropriate appliances is essential to managing ileostomy effectively. There are a plethora of options to choose from, including skin barriers and different pouching systems, so making decisions requires careful thought. Stoma size and shape, skin sensitivity, and lifestyle factors all impact the choice of appliances.

One-piece systems are straightforward, while two-piece systems allow for flexibility in changing pouches without removing the skin barrier. Recognizing the advantages and special characteristics of convex or flat barriers helps to address problems like retraction or irregular stomas. Additionally, researching innovations such as moldable wafers and pre-cut appliances helps to create a customized and practical solution for people overcoming ileostomy.

Upkeep And Handling

Maintenance and care form the cornerstone of successful ileostomy management, ensuring the longevity of appliances and the well-being of the individual. Regular skin inspection around the stoma is paramount to identify any signs of irritation, redness, or leakage.

Proper cleaning of the stoma and surrounding skin with mild, non-irritating products is essential for preventing infections and maintaining skin health. Adequate hydration is crucial, as it influences the consistency of stool output, impacting the performance of the pouching system. Education on proper disposal techniques and guidelines for changing the pouch at appropriate intervals contributes to a hygienic and comfortable experience. Moreover, staying vigilant about potential complications such as peristomal hernias or prolapsed stomas is vital for proactive management. In essence, meticulous maintenance and care practices are integral components in the holistic approach to conquering ileostomy and fostering an improved quality of life for those affected.

CHAPTER FOUR
DAILY MANAGEMENT TECHNIQUES

Overcoming Ileostomy necessitates a multifaceted strategy that includes daily self-management methods, appropriate stoma care, diet and nutrition, and hygiene habits. All of these components are critical to maintaining the health and well-being of those who have an ileostomy.

Techniques For Daily Management

Adopting these techniques helps people feel more in control and confident about managing their daily life with an ileostomy. Good daily management techniques are necessary for people with an ileostomy to maintain optimal health and adjust to changes in their digestive system.

These techniques include developing a routine that includes regular monitoring of stoma function, pouch changes, and skin inspection.

People with an ileostomy should also be taught how to recognize signs of complications like dehydration, blockages, or skin issues so that they can take prompt action.

Appropriate Stoma Management

The stoma, a surgically created opening in the abdomen through which waste is expelled, requires careful attention to maintain its health. Cleaning the stoma with mild soap and water during each pouch change helps prevent skin irritation and infections. A well-fitting ostomy pouch is necessary to ensure a secure and leak-free seal around the stoma.

Regular evaluation of the stoma's size and shape allows individuals to choose the most appropriate pouching system. Monitoring the color and consistency of the output is another important aspect of stoma care, as changes may indicate potential health issues that require medical attention.

By giving proper stoma care top priority, individuals can improve their overall well-being.

Nutrition And Diet

Diet and nutrition are critical to the successful management of an ileostomy. Patients should be informed about dietary choices that promote digestive health while reducing the risk of complications. A balanced diet consisting of a range of nutrient-rich foods is necessary to prevent nutritional deficiencies.

Since the small intestine absorbs vital nutrients, it is important to concentrate on easily digestible foods. Adequate fluid intake is critical to prevent dehydration, especially given the increased risk due to higher fluid loss from the stoma output. Fiber intake should be moderated to prevent complications like blockages, and foods that may cause gas or odor should be consumed in moderation.

Hygienic Habits

In order to prevent infections and maintain skin health, people with ileostomies must follow certain hygiene practices: wash their hands thoroughly before and after handling the ostomy pouch to reduce the chance of contamination; keep the skin around the stoma dry and clean to prevent irritation and breakdown; use gentle, fragrance-free cleansing products to prevent skin sensitivities; regularly check the peristomal skin for signs of redness, irritation, or infection to enable early intervention and prevent complications; use barrier creams or powders to maintain a healthy peristomal skin barrier; these measures not only improve the physical well-being of the individual, but they also have a positive psychological impact.

overcoming an ileostomy requires a comprehensive strategy that takes into account daily management methods, appropriate stoma care, diet and nutrition, and hygiene practices. These interrelated components are essential for people to adjust to the changes in their digestive system and live a happy and healthy life after surgery. By implementing these ideas into their daily routine, people can face the challenges of having an ileostomy with self-assurance and fortitude.

CHAPTER FIVE
OVERCOMING
CHALLENGES

Living with an ileostomy comes with its own set of difficulties that call for fortitude, flexibility, and a proactive approach. The main issues that people with ileostomies deal with are skin irritation and leakage. The stoma, which is a surgically made opening in the abdominal wall through which waste passes, requires close monitoring to avoid complications. Patients often use sophisticated ostomy appliances that have effective adhesive technology to prevent leaks. Patients can feel more secure and comfortable knowing that their pouching system is regularly checked and changed.

Furthermore, controlling skin irritation is essential for a good ileostomy experience. The sensitive skin around the stoma is prone to irritation from moisture and digestive enzymes. Using good hygiene practices, like cleaning and drying the peristomal skin thoroughly, is a critical step in avoiding skin problems. Adding skin barrier products and protective creams to the mix also helps to protect the skin from irritation, which improves general health and quality of life for ileostomy users.

Handling Skin Irritation And Leaks

For people living with an ileostomy, addressing skin irritation and leakage is critical.

Leakage, which can be a source of anxiety for ostomates, can be reduced with the use of modern ostomy appliances. Modern pouching systems are made to provide a secure seal, reducing the risk of leakage and providing comfort.

Consistent monitoring and prompt replacement of the pouching system are crucial practices to prevent leakage, enabling people living with an ileostomy to go about their daily lives without feeling embarrassed or uncomfortable.

Skin irritation, a common issue in the peristomal area, requires a comprehensive approach.

In addition to strict hygiene practices, people can investigate protective barriers and skin-friendly products designed specifically for ostomy care. These solutions act as a barrier against the harsh effects of moisture and digestive enzymes, fostering a healthy environment for the peristomal skin. By providing patients with information about proper skincare and access to cutting-edge products, patients can confidently navigate the challenges of skin irritation, improving their overall well-being and ability to adjust to life with an ileostomy.

Handling Ileostomy Odor

Effective odor management is critical to promoting a positive self-image and advancing social integration. The digestive process in the ileostomy produces effluent that can result in odorous output, which can negatively impact the patient's confidence and social interactions.

Odor management is an important part of ileostomy care, impacting both the physical and psychological well-being of individuals.

In the quest for odor control, people who have an ileostomy can employ a variety of tactics. Filter-equipped specialized pouching systems are made to neutralize and contain odors efficiently. Frequent replacements of the pouching system, strict hygiene regimens, and the application of deodorizing products help to reduce offensive odors. Dietary modifications, such as avoiding specific foods that are known to produce strong odors, can also be a useful part of odor management. By tackling the complex issue of odor control, people with an ileostomy can face everyday life with more assurance and a feeling of normalcy.

Traveling Despite Having An Ileostomy With Confidence

Traveling introduces a variety of factors, from changes in diet and time zones to variations in restroom accessibility, all of which can impact individuals with an ileostomy. In order to travel with confidence, ostomates must engage in proactive preparation and arm themselves with the necessary resources. Traveling with an ileostomy requires careful planning and consideration to ensure a seamless and confident experience.

Getting ready for the trip entails learning about destination-specific details like accessible restrooms and ostomy supplies. It's also important to pack an ostomy travel kit that includes extra pouching systems, skin care products, and any medications that may be needed in case of emergency. Finally, discreetly alerting airline personnel or appropriate authorities to your ileostomy can make your trip more comfortable by guaranteeing privacy and help when you need it.

A sense of community is fostered and ostomates are empowered to travel with confidence, broadening their horizons and embracing a fulfilling life beyond the limitations of their medical condition by sharing tips, advice, and success stories. When navigating the challenges of traveling with an ileostomy, individuals can draw on the experiences and insights of support groups or healthcare professionals.

CHAPTER SIX
MOVEMENT AND ACTIVITIES

Exercise and physical activity are important components of a healthy lifestyle for people with ileostomies. Regular exercise is necessary to keep the heart healthy, prevent obesity, and build muscle. However, people with ileostomies may find it difficult at first to adjust to their new situation. It is important that people speak with their healthcare providers to develop a customized exercise program that takes into account the particulars of living with an ileostomy.

Fear of complications from physical exertion is one of the main concerns for people who have an ileostomy. It is important to know the limitations and to gradually increase the intensity of physical activities. Low-impact exercises, like walking or gentle stretching, can help build confidence and assess one's physical capabilities.

As one gets more comfortable, they can gradually add more strenuous activities to their routine.

Managing An Ileostomy While Being Active

The physical and psychological aspects of maintaining an active lifestyle with an ileostomy must be addressed. Physical activity promotes better physical health and also has a positive impact on mental health. People who have an ileostomy frequently worry about the possible effects of exercise on their stoma, fearing leakage or other complications. In order to allay these worries, it is important to select the right kinds of activities and take the necessary precautions.

It is important to choose activities that are easy on the abdominal muscles and do not put excessive pressure on the stoma. Low-impact activities like swimming, cycling, or yoga can be great options. Using a supportive ostomy belt or wrap can also offer extra security and ease worries about the integrity of the stoma when exercising.

Finally, doing regular pelvic floor exercises can help improve control and stability around the stoma site.

Customizing Workout Programs

It is crucial to modify exercise regimens to meet the unique requirements of people who have an ileostomy in order to ensure safety and effectiveness. Variations in routines should take into account the patient's general health, the kind of surgery they have had, and any special guidelines or instructions from medical professionals. Patients should collaborate closely with healthcare providers, such as surgeons and ostomy nurses, in order to create a customized exercise regimen.

Combining aerobic, strength, and flexibility exercises can make for a well-rounded fitness regimen. Strength training builds muscle endurance, aerobic exercises improve cardiovascular health, and flexibility exercises improves joint mobility. To allow the body to adjust, it's important to start slowly and work your way up to more intense activities. It's also important to stay hydrated and to keep an eye out for any signs of strain or discomfort during exercise.

Recreational And Sports

It is possible and even very rewarding for people who want to live an active and fulfilling life to participate in sports and recreational activities with an ileostomy. Many sports can be modified to meet the needs of people who have an ileostomy, which promotes inclusion and empowerment.

However, people should approach sports and recreational activities with a thoughtful and cautious mindset, taking the necessary precautions to ensure a positive and safe experience.

Activities like swimming, golf, and hiking are generally well-tolerated by people with ileostomies. Swimming's buoyancy makes it a low-impact exercise option, and golf's slower pace allows for better control.

Hiking can be a great way to get some cardio exercise and connect with nature if done carefully and thoughtfully. It's important to be open and honest with healthcare providers about which sports and activities are best for each individual and their health.

overcoming obstacles after ileostomy requires accepting exercise and physical activity as essential elements of a healthy lifestyle.

Through appropriate exercise, customized routines, and participation in sports and leisure pursuits, people can overcome early obstacles and lead active, fulfilling lives after ileostomy. Individualized support from medical professionals and a gradual, flexible approach to physical activity also contribute to a positive experience, promoting mental and physical health.

CHAPTER SEVEN
NAVIGATING SOCIAL SITUATIONS

The journey to overcome ileostomy is complex and goes beyond the surgical procedure itself. One of the most important aspects of a person's life after ileostomy surgery is navigating social situations. This process necessitates a careful balancing act between preserving one's sense of normalcy and acclimating to the changes resulting from the surgical intervention. Social interactions can be difficult at first because people with ileostomy frequently struggle with issues related to body image and self-esteem. The ability to adjust and prosper in social settings is vital to the person's overall well-being.

When a person first starts to adjust to having an ileostomy, they might worry about how other people will perceive their changed body image. Learning about the stoma and related appliances is crucial to building self-confidence.

It is important to approach social situations with an optimistic attitude, stressing that having an ileostomy is a life-saving measure rather than a barrier to social interaction. Promoting open communication with friends, family, and coworkers can create a supportive environment, fostering understanding and empathy.

In addition, assimilating into social circles might necessitate deliberate preparation, like deciding which clothes to wear in order to cover or expose the ostomy pouch depending on how comfortable one is. Consulting support groups and mental health specialists can also help people develop coping strategies to deal with social situations effectively. As society's views change, promoting ileostomy awareness becomes a powerful tool for debunking myths and misconceptions and creating a welcoming environment for people with ostomies.

Speaking With Others

The key to overcoming ileostomy is effective communication because it promotes empathy and understanding between people who have and do not have ostomies. Honest and open discussion about the difficulties and adjustments following ileostomy surgery can close knowledge gaps and create a supportive community.

People should learn how to communicate effectively in order to express their needs, concerns, and experiences in a way that makes others feel heard and understood.

Providing accurate information about the surgical procedure, daily maintenance, and potential challenges helps dispel misconceptions and reduce stigma. Asking questions and having candid conversations with close friends, family, and coworkers creates an environment where people can share their experiences without feeling judged, which lays the groundwork for supportive relationships.

Moreover, nonverbal cues and body language are also forms of communication. Self-assurance in communicating can positively impact others' perceptions and reactions to one's ileostomy experience. Developing self-assurance in communication also contributes to the development of assertiveness, empowering people to set boundaries and speak up for themselves.

Mastering the art of communication empowers individuals with ileostomy to navigate social interactions with grace and resilience. In healthcare settings, effective communication with medical professionals is crucial for receiving optimal care. Patients with ileostomy must actively engage in discussions about their medical history, symptoms, and concerns in order for healthcare providers to be well-informed and able to tailor their care plans accordingly.

Closeness And Interactions

Overcoming ileostomy entails negotiating the complexities of intimacy and relationships, where the physical and emotional realms collide.

People who have ileostomy may struggle with issues of body image, self-worth, and rejection anxiety, all of which can negatively affect their capacity to form and sustain close relationships. Recognizing and resolving these issues is essential to promoting positive relationships and realizing a satisfying romantic life after surgery.

One of the most common issues in the area of intimacy is body image. People who have ileostomies may experience a change in their sense of self-worth and worry that their partners will find the stoma uncomfortable or unsightly. Overcoming these worries requires education and open communication. Partners should be made aware of the surgery, the reason for the stoma, and the fact that intimate relationships can resume after ileostomy.

Fostering a caring and understanding environment facilitates mutual reassurance and strengthens the emotional bond between partners.

In addition, it is imperative that people with ileostomies prioritize accepting and valuing their bodies for what they are. Developing self-assurance regarding one's physical appearance can have a positive impact on the dynamics of close relationships. Joining support groups or consulting a mental health professional can be helpful in managing body image concerns and fostering self-worth.

Taking Care Of Misconceptions And Stigma

In order to conquer ileostomy, it is necessary to address the stigma and misconceptions that the public has about ostomies. Stigmatization is frequently caused by ignorance, which results in prejudiced attitudes and discriminatory behavior. To address this problem, a multifaceted strategy that includes advocacy, education, and creating an inclusive environment is needed.

Education is key to eradicating myths surrounding ileostomy. Online and offline public awareness campaigns can accurately explain the surgical procedure, its goal, and what life is like with an ostomy. Working together with advocacy groups, community organizations, and healthcare providers is crucial to reaching a larger audience and challenging preconceived notions.

Promoting narratives that emphasize the accomplishments and resiliency of people with ileostomies is another way to combat stigma.

By sharing the successes, contributions, and life stories of people who have ostomies, we can dispel misconceptions and highlight the range of skills that people can acquire after surgery. Media representation and storytelling also serve as effective means of changing public opinion.

In addition, a supportive community that accepts and elevates people with ileostomies is essential to overcoming stigma.

Online and offline support groups offer a forum for people to share stories, receive encouragement, and feel like they belong. Policy changes that safeguard the rights of people with ostomies should be the goal of advocacy campaigns.

overcoming ileostomy involves more than just surgery; it also involves navigating the complexities of social dynamics, communication, intimacy, and the fight against stigma.

Through advocacy, education, and resilience, people with ileostomy can lead fulfilling lives and help advance the larger movement of de-stigmatizing ostomies in society.

CHAPTER EIGHT
CONSIDERATIONS FOR WORK AND CAREERS

Living with an ileostomy comes with a special set of difficulties, especially when it comes to work and career planning. People with ileostomies frequently worry about workplace adjustments, career planning, and striking a delicate balance between work and health.

Navigating A Career After An Ileostomy

When it comes to career planning, people with ileostomies have to take into account their skill set, professional objectives, and the physical demands of the career path they have chosen. Some professions can be difficult to work in because of the nature of the work or the workplace; in these situations, people may need to reevaluate their goals and look into other options that are more in line with their abilities and health condition. Communication with coworkers and employers is essential during this process because it helps people understand the difficulties an ileostomy may cause while showcasing one's dedication and ability to make a significant contribution to the workplace.

Workplace Perquisites

In order to create a welcoming and supportive work environment for people with ileostomies, it is imperative that employers and HR departments have a thorough understanding of the unique needs of workers with ileostomies, acknowledging that accommodations may differ based on the nature of the job. Common modifications that can greatly improve the quality of life for people with ileostomies include ergonomic seating arrangements, accessible restrooms, and flexible break times. Additionally, cultivating an inclusive and sensitive work culture fosters a more accepting environment where employees feel comfortable sharing their needs and requesting the accommodations they require.

Finding A Work-Health Balance

For people who have an ileostomy, finding a delicate balance between work and health is a constant concern. The physical and emotional demands of the workplace can have an impact on one's health, and vice versa.

The prevention of burnout and potential health complications can be achieved by prioritizing self-care and setting boundaries. Regular check-ups and open communication with healthcare providers are crucial elements of managing one's health effectively. Employers can also support employees in finding a balance between work and health by fostering a culture that values well-being, encourages breaks when needed, and offers flexibility when handling medical appointments or unforeseen health-related issues.

managing work and career issues when one has an ileostomy necessitates a careful and comprehensive approach. Career planning entails reevaluating goals and making any necessary adjustments to align with one's health condition. Workplace accommodations are essential in fostering an inclusive and supportive environment, acknowledging the unique needs of individuals with an ileostomy. Balancing work and health is a continuous process that calls for open communication, self-care, and cooperation between employers and employees. With a thorough understanding of these ideas, people with an ileostomy can pursue rewarding careers while putting their health and well-being first.

CHAPTER NINE
UPCOMING DEVELOPMENTS AND STUDIES

The future of overcoming ileostomy entails a multimodal strategy that combines state-of-the-art discoveries with ongoing research initiatives. Technological developments are critical to improving the quality of life for people who have an ileostomy; scientists are currently investigating new materials for stoma appliances that are more comfortable, discrete, and friendly to the skin. Additionally, advanced ostomy pouching systems with built-in sensors to track parameters like pH levels and output consistency are being developed with the goal of giving users access to real-time data so they can better manage their condition.

Research is being conducted in the field of surgical interventions to improve long-term outcomes, minimize complications, and shorten recovery times.

Robotic-assisted surgeries are becoming more popular as a means of improving precision and reducing invasiveness.

Researchers are also exploring the possibility of using regenerative medicine to encourage tissue regeneration and healing around the stoma site, which could lead to improvements in the overall functionality and durability of ileostomy sites.

Patient-centric research is becoming more and more popular, emphasizing a comprehensive understanding of the psychosocial impact of having an ileostomy. Research on the psychological aspects of body image, self-esteem, and the social implications of an altered body function may be explored in the future.

The goal of this all-encompassing approach is to inform the creation of support networks and mental health interventions that are specifically designed to meet the needs of individuals with ileostomies.

Improvements In Ostomy Care

In order to improve comfort, adherence, and overall satisfaction for users of ileostomies, manufacturers are investing in research to create products that offer enhanced wear time, leak prevention, and odor control.

Additionally, biocompatible materials are being explored to minimize skin irritation and allergies, addressing common challenges faced by ileostomy patients. These advancements in ostomy care are crucial to the quality of life for people living with ileostomies.

Smart ostomy appliances with Bluetooth connectivity and mobile applications enable users to track and manage their output, receive timely alerts for pouch changes, and access personalized care information. These technological advancements not only help improve self-management but also make remote monitoring by healthcare professionals possible, promoting a more proactive approach to care. The integration of smart technologies into ostomy care is a noteworthy trend.

Apart from new product developments, improvements in stoma care nursing are also leading to better patient outcomes. Healthcare professionals can benefit from specialized training programs that optimize stoma site assessment, personalized education, and continuous support. This guarantees that patients with ileostomies receive individualized care that is in line with their specific needs and challenges.

New Technologies

A notable development in ileostomy care is the application of artificial intelligence (AI), which can analyze data from wearable devices like smart ostomy pouches to predict and prevent potential problems like leaks or skin irritation.

By taking a proactive approach, this can significantly lower the frequency of complications and improve the overall quality of life for ileostomy patients. Emerging technologies are changing the landscape of ileostomy management by providing new possibilities for improved functionality and increased patient autonomy.

In the context of ileostomy care, telemedicine is becoming more and more relevant by offering remote access to medical professionals for consultation and support. Telemonitoring solutions and virtual clinics allow for timely interventions, reducing the need for frequent in-person visits, which not only improves patient convenience but also guarantees ongoing monitoring and the ability to modify care plans in accordance with individual needs.

Customized stoma appliances, belts, and accessories can be made to precisely fit the unique anatomy of each patient, improving adherence and reducing discomfort.

This personalized approach represents a shift towards patient-centered care, acknowledging the variety of anatomical variations among ileostomy patients.

3D printing technology is making significant advancements in the customization of ostomy products.

Patient Involvement And Advocacy

The key to conquering ileostomy is patient advocacy and involvement, which highlights the significance of enabling people with a lived experience to actively engage in their care journey. Advocacy groups and organizations are essential in increasing awareness, advancing education, and fighting for the rights of ileostomy patients. They provide a supportive and community environment and provide a forum for people to share their experiences, struggles, and victories.

Beyond support groups, patient involvement includes active participation in research, policy development, and decision-making related to healthcare. Incorporating ileostomy patients' perspectives into the design and assessment of healthcare interventions guarantees that solutions are customized to their individual needs and preferences.

Patient-reported outcomes are increasingly acknowledged as important indicators of treatment success, offering insights into the comprehensive effects of interventions on people's lives.

Furthermore, social media and digital platforms have become effective instruments for patient advocacy. Online communities offer a forum for people to interact, exchange resources, and obtain information. Advocates and influencers for patients use their platforms to spread information, combat stigma, and support a positive story about having an ileostomy.

the ongoing journey to conquer ileostomy is made possible by concerted efforts in future innovations and research, advances in ostomy care, emerging technologies, and patient advocacy and involvement. By adopting a holistic and patient-centered approach, the healthcare landscape is evolving to provide more individualized, efficient, and empowering solutions for people living with ileostomies.

CHAPTER TEN
INSPIRING SUCCESS STORIES

Inspirational tales of ileostomy success emphasize the fortitude and tenacity of people who have overcome the difficulties related to this medical procedure. These stories typically revolve around people who have recovered control over their lives after the initial shock and adjustment period. Success stories may address emotional, physical, or social aspects. They also illuminate the coping mechanisms that ileostomy patients utilize, stressing the value of optimism, support systems, and accepting a new normal. Finally, these tales offer hope to those who are experiencing similar situations by demonstrating that life after ileostomy can be both manageable and rewarding.

Individual Testimonials

By sharing their personal stories, people help others better understand the psychological and emotional aspects of living with an ileostomy, which promotes empathy and dispels stigmas associated with this medical condition. Testimonials frequently touch on the initial fears, anxieties, and misconceptions surrounding ileostomy surgery, giving readers a glimpse into the raw and unfiltered reality of the process. Personally, narratives offer an intimate and firsthand account of the experiences people go through when dealing with ileostomy.

These narratives delve into the emotional rollercoaster of acceptance, the difficulties of adjusting to a new lifestyle, and the evolution of self-identity.

Ileostomy Champions' Profiles

These profiles of ileostomy champions highlight people who have not only accepted their new reality but have also taken on the roles of educators and advocates within the ileostomy community. These champions frequently use their experiences to dispel social stigmas associated with ostomies, educate others, and shed light on the life-changing journeys these people have taken, from the initial challenges to the empowerment that comes with accepting their ileostomy. By taking on these roles, these champions help to dispel myths about ileostomy, promote inclusivity, and foster a more accepting and supportive community.

Overcoming Obstacles

In the context of ileostomy, the idea of triumphs over challenges embodies the multitude of challenges that people encounter and overcome in their lives after surgery. These challenges can range from managing the physical aspects of the stoma and pouch system to addressing psychological and social challenges.

Examining these triumphs highlights the adaptability and resilience of patients with ileostomies. Examples of these triumphs include overcoming social stigma, managing body image issues, and successfully reintegrating into the workplace and social environments.

CONCLUSION

the journey of conquering ileostomy is a complex and multifaceted one that involves a profound shift in physical, emotional, and social dimensions of an individual's life.

Through inspiring success stories, personal testimonials, profiles of ileostomy champions, and triumphs over challenges, a comprehensive understanding of the transformative nature of the ileostomy experience emerges.

These narratives collectively emphasize the importance of resilience, support networks, and a positive mindset in navigating the challenges posed by ileostomy surgery.

The power of personal stories and the advocacy of champions play a crucial role in dispelling myths, fostering empathy, and promoting a more inclusive and understanding society for individuals living with an ileostomy.

As medical advancements continue to improve the quality of life for ileostomy patients, these narratives serve as a testament to the human spirit's ability to triumph over adversity and redefine what it means to live a fulfilling and meaningful life post-ileostomy.